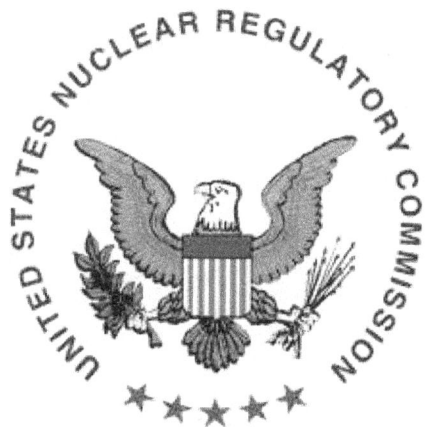

ALLEGATION PROGRAM

2005 ANNUAL TRENDS REPORT

CONTENTS

EXECUTIVE SUMMARY

Management Directive 8.8, "Management of Allegations," requires the Agency Allegations Advisor to prepare an annual report for the Executive Director for Operations that provides an analysis of allegation trends. This annual report fulfills that commitment by providing national, regional, and site specific trend analyses.

There were also several agency activities in 2005 involving the Allegation Program that warrant mention in this report, including new guidance prepared by the staff in the area of safety conscious work environment. After appreciable stakeholder involvement and endorsement by the Committee to Review Generic Requirements, Regulatory Issue Summary 2005-18, "Guidance for Establishing and Maintaining a Safety Conscious Work Environment," was issued on August 25, 2005 in accordance with direction provided by the Commission in Staff Requirements Memorandum (SRM) SECY-04-0111. In the same SRM, the Commission also directed the staff to enhance the Reactor Oversight Process (ROP) to more fully address safety culture. This report summaries the significant progress achieved in 2005 on this initiative as well. ROP enhancements included changes to the Safety Conscious Work Environment cross-cutting area and related inspection documents. In addition, the allegations staff continues to implement the agency sponsored Alternative Dispute Resolution Program for discrimination allegations and has made revisions to the Allegation Program based on feedback during the pilot phase of the program. Lastly, an Allegation Guidance Memorandum was developed in 2005 implementing Commission direction to severely limit the release of security-related information to the public, including allegers. To address concerns that these changes have the potential to impact the public's willingness to raise security-related concerns to the Nuclear Regulatory Commission (NRC), the staff continues to work with the Office of Nuclear Security and Incident Response to define further guidance on the level of information that is appropriate to provide to allegers in response to security-related allegations.

With regard to allegation trends, as the figure to the right indicates, from calendar year 2001 through 2005 the number of allegations received by the NRC has remained steady with incremental annual increases in the reactor area from 2003 to 2005. With the exception of Region III, increases were seen in each region. Significant contributors to the decrease in allegations received in Region III since 2002 included the transfer of oversight responsibility for two large fuel cycle facilities from Region III to Region II; the addition of another Agreement State; and the completion of the extended shutdown at the Davis-Besse plant. The number of security-related issues increased in 2005 and again, comprised the largest percentage of alleged concerns received in the calendar year. The increase is attributed to concerns raised during a national broadcast regarding security at research and test reactors.

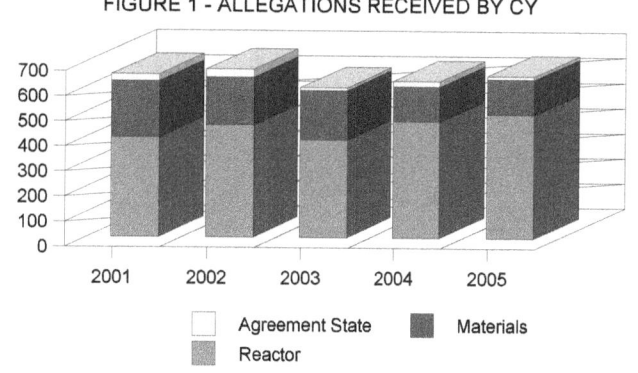

FIGURE 1 - ALLEGATIONS RECEIVED BY CY

For some licensees, the NRC received allegations in numbers that warranted additional analysis. In preparing this report, a 5-year history of allegations was reviewed for reactor and material licensees and vendors to identify adverse trends. The analysis focused on allegations that originated from onsite sources to help inform the NRC's review of the safety conscious work environment.[1] The staff identified 15 reactor sites for a more in-depth review: Salem/Hope Creek, Browns Ferry Unit 1, Palo Verde Units 1, 2 & 3, Susquehanna Units 1 & 2, St. Lucie Units 1 & 2, Oyster Creek, Point Beach Units 1 & 2, Byron Units 1 & 2, Callaway, Millstone Units 2 & 3, Sequoyah Units 1 & 2, Seabrook, Shearon Harris Units 1 & 2, Dresden Units 2 & 3, and Comanche Peak Units 1 & 2. Allegation trends at each of these sites are discussed in the report. In summary, the trends either did not suggest a weakening safety conscious work environment or the licensee is taking steps to address trends and the NRC is monitoring those activities. No materials licensees or vendors were the subject of allegations at a level that warranted additional analysis.

---

[1] The total number of allegations received concerning reactor licensees from all sources, as well as other information concerning the Allegation Program, can be found on the NRC's public website at http://www.nrc.gov/what-we-do/regulatory/allegations-resp.html.

OVERVIEW OF SIGNIFICANT PROGRAM ACTIVITIES

Several significant agency activities took place in 2005 that affect the Allegation Program and warrant discussion in this report. Guidance for establishing and maintaining a safety conscious work environment was issued in accordance with direction provided by the Commission in Staff Requirements Memorandum (SRM) SECY-04-0111, dated August 30, 2004. In this SRM, the Commission also directed the staff to enhance the Reactor Oversight Process to more fully address safety culture, while continuing to monitor industry and foreign efforts in this area. Significant progress was achieved in 2005 on the agency's safety culture initiative. In addition, the allegations staff continues to implement the agency sponsored Alternative Dispute Resolution process for discrimination allegations and has made revisions to the program based on feedback during the pilot phase of the program. Lastly, the allegations staff responded to initial guidance from the Commission regarding the release of security-related information to the public. Consistent with more recent direction from the Commission in SRM-SECY-05-0082, the allegation staff continues to work with the Office of Nuclear Security and Incident Response to develop additional guidance on the level of information that is appropriate to provide to allegers in response to security-related allegations. These areas are discussed in more detail below.

Safety Conscious Work Environment and Safety Culture

The Commission directed the staff in March 2003 to prepare further guidance for licensees on establishing a safety conscious work environment (SCWE), that is, an environment where employees in the nuclear industry are encouraged to raise safety concerns to their employers or the Nuclear Regulatory Commission (NRC) without fear of retaliation, and where concerns are effectively addressed. The Commission's expectation that licensees establish and maintain a SCWE was outlined in a May 19, 1996, Policy Statement, "Freedom of Employees in the Nuclear Industry to Raise Safety Concerns Without Fear of Retaliation." However, the guidance provided by the policy statement is very broad, and, with the staff continuing to see SCWE concerns at a variety of facilities, the Commission directed the staff to provide further guidance to the industry in this area.

In the Fall of 2003, the staff formed a working group and outlined a draft SCWE guidance document based on the content of the 1996 Policy Statement. This outline was published in the *Federal Register* for comment and was the basis for discussion at a public meeting on February 19, 2004. While most of the stakeholders at the meeting, including representatives from the industry and whistleblower advocates, agreed on the content of such a document, there were many comments concerning the format, potential inappropriate use of the guidance, and the appropriateness of the NRC issuing such guidance.

Coincident with these comments, the Commission requested through ticketed correspondence that the staff provide recommended actions regarding agency guidance in the areas of SCWE and safety culture. In the paper that addressed the Commission's request, the staff sought further guidance from the Commission on whether to continue to pursue issuance of the guidance document, in light of the comments received. In SRM-SECY-04-0111, the Commission directed the staff to continue its efforts to issue the guidance, following a brief comment period. In October 2004, the Office of Enforcement (OE) staff published in the *Federal Register* for comment the full guidance document, which incorporated many of the suggestions made as a result of the first public comment period. The staff reviewed all comments received and made significant revisions in response to comments that the guidance was too prescriptive and that much of the guidance was applicable only to larger facilities. The

Committee to Review Generic Requirements endorsed issuance of the guidance in June of 2005, and Regulatory Issue Summary 2005-018, "Guidance for Establishing and Maintaining a Safety Conscious Work Environment," was issued on August 25, 2005.

Regarding the related area of safety culture, the Commission approved, also in SRM-SECY-04-0111, the following actions: (1) continue to monitor industry efforts to assess safety culture and ensure that the Commission remains informed of industry efforts and progress; (2) enhance the Reactor Oversight Process (ROP) treatment of cross-cutting issues to more fully address safety culture; (3) include as part of enhanced inspection activities for plants in the degraded cornerstone column of the reactor oversight action matrix, a determination of the need for a specific evaluation of the licensee's safety culture and a method for conducting such an evaluation; and (4) continue to monitor developments by foreign regulators in this area. The Commission emphasized the need for inspector training in this area and stakeholder involvement in the process of enhancing the ROP.

In order to address the Commission's direction, the OE staff formed a safety culture working group comprised of members representing the Offices of Nuclear Reactor Regulation (NRR), Research (RES), Nuclear Material Safety and Safeguards (NMSS), and OE who have expertise in human factors, SCWE, or inspection. The working group was supplemented by regional inspectors who provided their expertise in development of the approach to enhance the ROP. In addition, OE formed a Safety Culture Steering Committee which is comprised of management representatives from OE, NRR, RES, NMSS, and Region II to provide policy direction to the working group and review working group draft products.

In the fall of 2005, the working group, along with internal and external stakeholders, held a series of public meetings during which an approach to addressing the Commission's direction to more fully address safety culture was developed. The approach is consistent with the ROP framework and involves aligning the current cross-cutting areas with what is important to safety culture. As such, inspector findings of performance deficiencies identified under the ROP will be evaluated to determine whether the components of safety culture (i.e, cross-cutting aspects) contributed to the deficiency. The approach is graded, in that as plant performance deteriorates and plants move across the ROP action matrix from the "Licensee Response" column to the "Multiple/Repetitive Degraded Cornerstone" column, NRC inspection and oversight of the site's safety culture appropriately becomes more intrusive. The approach also involves providing more defined assessment criteria for the Safety Conscious Work Environment cross-cutting area and provides that if a plant is determined to have a substantive cross-cutting area for three consecutive plant assessments, the NRC may engage the licensee with respect to safety culture, including requesting that the site conduct an assessment of safety culture.

The staff is in the final stages of drafting revisions to several of the baseline, special, and supplemental reactor oversight inspection procedures, as well as other documents that guide the staff's assessment and documentation of findings, to more fully address the area of safety culture. Initial implementation of the revisions will begin in July 2006. In addition, the staff is developing training for the NRC staff regarding safety culture and the changes to the inspection process. This training will also include additional guidance for inspectors in the area of safety conscious work environment. The staff intends to train inspectors on the revised process before July 2006. Training for new inspectors with regard to the enhanced ROP and safety culture will be developed by the end of 2006.

Consistent with the Commission's direction, the staff has also continued to monitor industry and international efforts in the area of safety culture. For example, the staff observed two Institute of Nuclear Power Operations (INPO) plant evaluations which included safety culture assessments and used industry and international attributes of safety culture to inform the NRC's development of safety culture components. With regard to foreign developments in safety culture, the working group continues to collect information on safety culture efforts from foreign regulators, the International Atomic Energy Agency, and the Nuclear Energy Agency. The staff reviews such documents to determine their potential usefulness in the agency's safety culture initiatives.

The staff intends to provide the Commission with a more detailed status of the staff's efforts in this area in a Commission paper in mid-2006.

Alternative Dispute Resolution for Discrimination Allegations

In October 2004, the staff implemented a pilot Alternative Dispute Resolution (ADR) program which included the opportunity for using ADR early in the allegation process in cases of alleged discrimination, before the NRC conducts its investigation of the allegation. This allows additional opportunity for the parties to resolve their differences outside of the normal regulatory framework. Early-ADR involves the use of a neutral third party to facilitate discussion and timely settlement of the discrimination concern in an effort to minimize potential negative impact on the SCWE at the facility involved. At any time, either party can exit the ADR process and, if the alleger still wants to pursue the discrimination matter, the option of an investigation by the NRC remains. The staff's policy under the Early-ADR pilot program is not to pursue an investigation or subsequent enforcement of discrimination findings which have been settled through this process.

From the initiation of the pilot program in October 2004, through the end of calender year 2005, 24 allegers and their employers, of the 95 that were offered Early-ADR, have agreed to mediate. Mediation resulted in 8 settlement agreements between the alleger and the licensee (6 of the 24 are still in progress). The OE staff is continuing to monitor this program with regard to the number of cases where Early-ADR is pursued, the number of cases that settle, and indications of the effect of Early-ADR on the SCWE at the involved facilities.

In October 2005, the NRC staff held a public meeting to discuss stakeholder comments on the Early-ADR process. Feedback during the meeting was primarily positive with regard to the effectiveness of the Early-ADR program. However, as a result of feedback received, the staff has identified several initiatives that will be undertaken to improve the process including: (1) enhancing the type and amount of information shared between the parties prior to mediation; (2) clarifying the process for handling technical safety issues raised by the alleger; (3) providing information to the public on the number of Early-ADR offers, meditations, and settlements; and (4) providing additional orientation to ADR mediators regarding the NRC's process and regulations in the area of discrimination. Stakeholder feedback received and experience in processing Early-ADR cases has provided insight regarding additional potential enhancements to the program including: (1) more timely responses of the parties where Early-ADR is offered and, (2) ensuring appropriate representation of the licensee by individuals who are familiar with the issue and authorized to make decisions regarding any settlement.

As stated above, the primary objective of Early-ADR is to minimize potential negative impact on the safety conscious work environment. The Office of Enforcement recently evaluated the effectiveness of the program to assess its progress toward achieving the objective. Based upon the evaluation, the staff believes that voluntary dispute resolution by the parties using the communication opportunities afforded in Early-ADR can stem the inherent damage such disputes have on the SCWE more quickly than an investigation; however, there is no objective indication that Early-ADR has had an immediate positive impact on any particular facility's work environment. Indications of positive improvements may be limited to facilities that have successfully used ADR more than once and developed an improved environment over the long term. The staff concluded that, to date, the information available indicates that the assumed benefits of the Early-ADR process, including decreased costs and the impact on the SCWE, warrant continued use of Early-ADR in the Allegation Program. A more detailed assessment of the pilot program will be provided in a Commission paper.

Implementation of Guidance Regarding Release of Security-Related Information

Because of recent concerns about the release of information related to potential security vulnerabilities at licensed facilities, the Commission directed the staff, in SRM-SECY-04-0002, to no longer make certain types of security-related information available to the public. Although allegation correspondence is not normally made public, the potential does exist that correspondence to allegers and licensees that could reveal potential security-related vulnerabilities could be unnecessarily released.

In 2005, the staff drafted guidance concerning the marking and control of security-related allegation material (which was subsequently issued in March of 2006). The guidance incorporated the recommendations of the task group on Sensitive Unclassified Non-Safeguards Information with regard to the marking and control of security-related material. Consistent with the Commission's direction, the guidance reflects that only the stated concern can be provided to the alleger. Except in cases where there is adequate justification, letters to allegers raising security-related information no longer provide information on the agency's inspection activity or actions taken to resolve the allegation. In such cases where more information is proposed to be released, coordination with the Office of Nuclear Security and Incident Response (NSIR) is required. Because this marks a significant change in the amount of information provided to allegers on security-related issues, the Agency Allegations Advisor has been monitoring the potential effects of this guidance on the willingness of individuals to raise security allegations to the NRC. The staff continues to receive negative feedback from allegers and other external stakeholders regarding this practice and recently has noted an increase in the use of media outlets and other more public venues to raise such concerns, prompting a more public response by the agency. Although security-related allegations continue to be a major contributor in the allegations received by the NRC, even increasing in 2005 compared to the prior year, the staff continues to look for improved ways to protect sensitive information while still being responsive to allegers. In particular, in accordance with the Commission's more recent direction in SRM-SECY-05-0082, "Assessment Process for the Security Cornerstone of the Reactor Oversight process," to provide more security-related information via the ROP, the staff is coordinating with NSIR to define further guidance concerning the level of detail which can appropriately be provided to allegers in response to security-related allegations. The staff will work to develop an Allegation Guidance Memorandum to provide such guidance during 2006.

TRENDS IN ALLEGATIONS

The NRC monitors both technical and discrimination allegations to discern trends or marked increases that might prompt the NRC to question the licensee as to the causes of such changes or trends. In preparing this report, a 5-year history of allegations received was reviewed for reactor and material licensees and vendors. The staff focused on those allegations that have the potential to provide insights into the SCWE at a given facility, that is, those allegations submitted by current or former licensee or contractor employees or by anonymous sources that indicate unwillingness to raise safety concerns internally. The staff performs an analysis of recent allegation activity twice a year in support of the ROP mid-cycle and end-of-cycle assessments. In addition, an analysis for a particular site or licensee may be performed whenever allegations or inspection findings indicate that such an analysis is warranted.

The staff also conducts reviews to identify national trends for reactor and materials allegations received, shifts in users of the NRC Allegation Program, and the impact of Allegation Program implementation on the workload in the regions, NRR and NMSS. These trends are discussed in the following section.

National Trends

National trends are of interest because they provide general information to the staff concerning the impact of external factors, plant events, and industry efforts to improve the SCWE at NRC licensed facilities. In addition, they are useful developing budget and planning assumptions to support future agency and allegation program needs. Figure 1 below shows that the 5-year national trend in allegation receipt has remained steady with incremental annual increases in the reactor area from 2003 to 2005.

FIGURE 1 - ALLEGATIONS RECEIVED BY CY

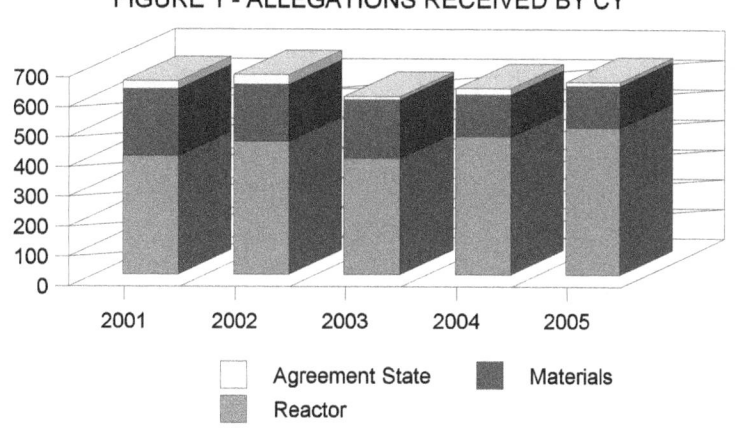

As each allegation can include multiple concerns, the number of concerns received provides more specific information with regard to staff effort needed for appropriate response. The trend in the total number of concerns received has paralleled the trend of total allegation receipt over the last five years; that is, the number of concerns received at operating power reactor facilities over the last five years has increased in all regions except one, and the number of materials issues received in every region has decreased. The volume of concerns received in Region I trended upward between 2003 and 2005. The increase in reactor issues during this time frame can be largely attributed to the identification of a significant SCWE concern at a Region I site. Additionally, the responsibility for oversight of all Region II materials licensees was transferred to Region I in 2003, and in 2004, several Region I reactor sites underwent contract negotiations or reorganizations. The volume of concerns in Region II has also trended upward for the last several years. The upward trend in reactor concerns at Region II since 2002 is likely due to plant specific occurrences related to construction activities at one reactor facility, and an increasing number of security concerns at several Region II reactor facilities in 2005. The number of concerns received in Region III over the past five years peaked in 2002, but has decreased steadily from 2003 to 2005. A significant contributor to the decrease in allegations received at Region III since 2002 was the transfer of oversight responsibility for two large fuel cycle facilities from Region III to Region II in 2003. Also in 2003, another state in the Region III geographical area achieved Agreement State status, wherein materials licensee allegations that would formerly have been processed by the NRC are now addressed by the Agreement State. Events that have also contributed to the reduction in Region III allegations were the resolution of union/strike issues at one plant and the end of the extended shutdown of another. The number of concerns received in Region IV fluctuated from 2001 through 2005, generally at lower totals than the other regions, but did increase notably from 2004 to 2005. This increase can largely be attributed to one multi-plant site. Overall, there has been an increase in the number of concerns received at operating power reactor facilities over the last five years in all regions except for Region III. In contrast, the number of materials issues has declined over the five-year period in every region.

Reactor Licensee Trends

To provide further insight into areas in which the NRC is spending resources on reactor-related allegation follow-up, Figure 2 below depicts the twelve functional areas that represent approximately 80 percent of the issues received nationwide in 2005.[2]

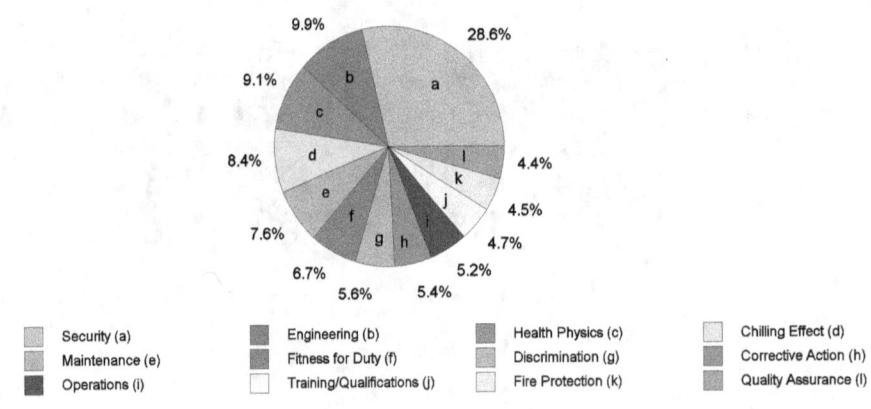

FIGURE 2 - REACTOR ISSUES NATIONWIDE 2005

Security (a)	Engineering (b)	Health Physics (c)	Chilling Effect (d)
Maintenance (e)	Fitness for Duty (f)	Discrimination (g)	Corrective Action (h)
Operations (i)	Training/Qualifications (j)	Fire Protection (k)	Quality Assurance (l)

[2]Few concerns were received in the areas representing the 20 percent not depicted in Figure 2. These areas include Access Authorization, Chemistry, Civil/Structural, Construction, Electrical, Emergency Planning, Employee Concerns Programs, Environmental, Environmental Qualification, Falsification, Fatigue/Overtime, Industrial Safety, Inservice Testing, Instrumentation & Control, Licensing, Mechanical, Non-destructive Evaluation, Other, Procurement, Radwaste, Safeguards, Safety Culture, and Wrongdoing.

As indicated in the pie chart, security issues comprised the largest percentage of alleged concerns received in 2005. Since the terrorist attacks of September 11, 2001, security-related concerns continue to represent the greatest percentage of concerns received, and in 2005 in particular, the program saw a 56 percent increase in security-related concerns. In previous years, increases were attributable to concerns about the effectiveness with which licensees implemented new NRC Security Orders. Licensees were required to be compliant with those orders, issued in 2003, by October 2004. More recently, a sharp increase in the number of security-related concerns was noted in association with a national broadcast in October 2005 regarding security at research and test reactors. In a public response, the NRC noted that based on the agency's review of those observations, a continuing review of site-specific security enhancements, and knowledge of low potential risks associated with such small quantities of radioactive material, the Nation's research and test reactors remain safe and secure.

Assertions related to "chilling effect" or a "chilled" work environment in which individuals fear retaliation or are discouraged from raising safety concerns, has trended upward overall in the last five years, although the number of issues received in this area has declined from a peak in 2003. While positive industry accomplishments in the SCWE area are believed to have contributed to the decrease in the receipt of "chilling effect" concerns after 2003, the recent upward trend (25 percent increase between 2004 and 2005) may reflect an increasing awareness of SCWE concepts by the nuclear workforce due to increased industry focus in this area, media interest concerning increased NRC focus in this area at some sites, as well as recent guidance made publically available by the NRC (i.e., Regulatory Issue Summary 2005-018, "Guidance for Establishing and Maintaining a Safety Conscious Work Environment," issued in August 2005). An increase in the number of sites where potential chilled work environment issues have been identified is also indicative of increased workforce awareness of SCWE concepts.

Regarding the distribution in the four regional offices and NRR of the same twelve areas illustrated in Figure 2, notable changes from 2004 to 2005 include: (1) a significant increase in the percentage of issues that relate to security in Region II and NRR. The increase in NRR was primarily due to the public broadcast regarding research and test reactors discussed above and the increase in Region II was due to a series of security-related allegations at a few reactor sites; (2) an increase in the percentage of health physics issues in Region II, primarily due to one circumstance at one Region II site; and (3) an increase in the number of engineering concerns in Region IV primarily due to specific incidents at two sites.

Materials Licensee Trends

Because of the many different types of materials licensees and because the activities performed by materials licensees are not as homogeneous as those performed by reactor licensees, a comparison of the types of issues received does not produce meaningful results. For insights into the areas in which the NRC is spending resources on materials-related allegations, the following chart depicts the eight materials licensee types from which approximately 80 percent of the issues have been received nationwide.[3]

FIGURE 3 - MATERIALS LICENSEE TYPES NATIONWIDE 2005

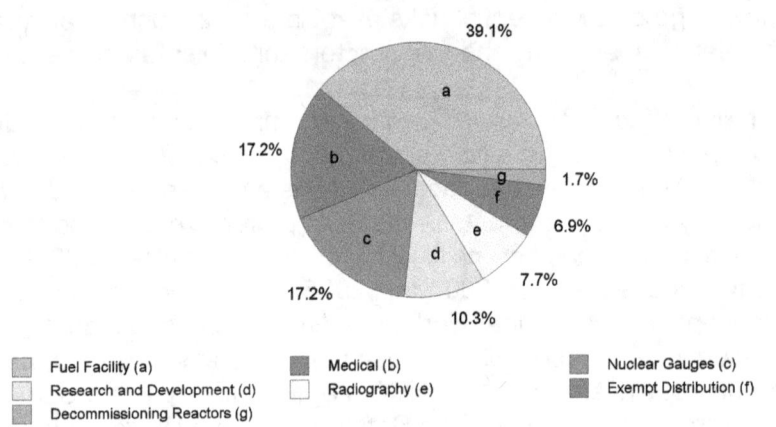

Notable changes in the distribution of materials-related allegation issues received nationally include an increasing trend in the number of issues related to fuel facilities since 2003, with a notable increase from 2004 to 2005. Notwithstanding the recent upward trend, the number of issues received related to fuel facilities from 2003 to 2005 is considerably smaller than those received in 2001 and 2002. The increase from 2004 to 2005 was largely attributable to a number of issues received at one fuel facility following a specific event, a change in management expectations regarding procedural adherence, and a planned workforce reduction in Fall 2005. There is a decreasing trend in the number of medical and radiography issues received in the last five years. An analysis of the data indicates no notable reason(s) for the decreases. In addition, the functional area of exempt distribution was one of the primary contributors to the allegations received in the materials area, primarily due to concerns received regarding the sale of products on the internet containing exempt quantities of radioactive material.

In the regions and program offices, notable changes include a sharp decrease in the number of decommissioning reactor allegations in Region I from 2004 to 2005 coinciding with the cessation of decommissioning activities at two sites. In addition, the number of allegations received related to decommissioning reactors in Region IV increased significantly from 2004 to 2005, primarily due to the receipt of an allegation regarding one facility with numerous concerns.

---

[3]Few concerns were received for the materials licensee types representing the 20 percent not depicted in Figure 3. These licensee types include Decommissioning Materials, General Licensee, Irradiators, Nuclear Pharmacies, Other, Transportation, Uranium Recovery, and Waste Disposal.

Source Trends

Figure 4 below provides a breakdown of 99 percent of the sources for reactors and materials allegations received in the last three years.[4] The data indicates that the distribution of source categories remained steady in the 2003 to 2005 time frame. That is, the primary sources of allegations continue to be licensee (or former licensee) employees and contractor (or former contractor) employees. It follows that the percentage of reactors and materials allegations from other sources has also remained largely unchanged for the last three years. One notable change in the data was the indication of the news media as a more prominent source of allegations in 2005. This was primarily due to a series of allegations in association with the October 2005 national broadcast about security at research and test reactors discussed previously.

FIGURE 4 - ALLEGATIONS BY SOURCE CATEGORY

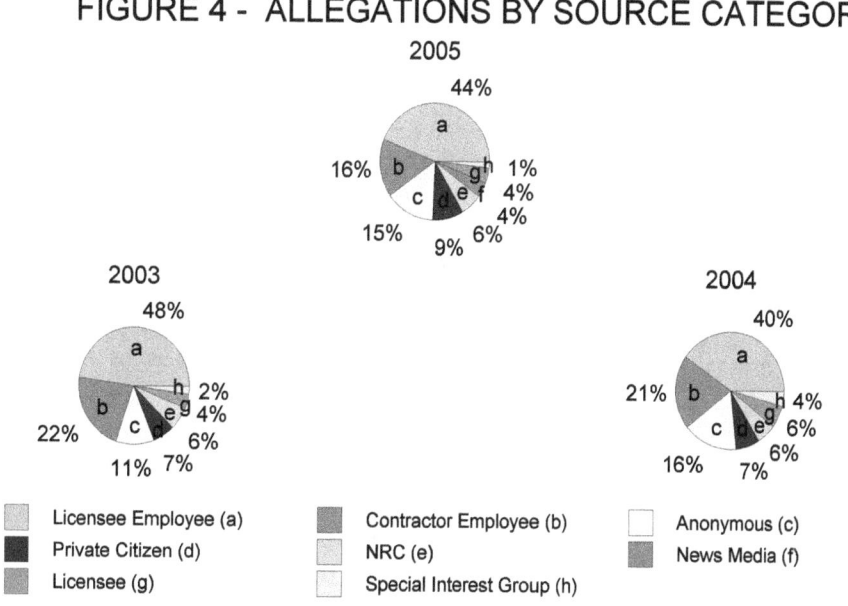

In comparing the sources of materials allegations to those of reactor allegations over the past few years, consistently the largest source for both are licensee (or former licensee) employees. It is worth noting, however, contractor employees are a less prevalent source of materials-related allegations while private citizens are a more prevalent source. This is understandable given that materials licensees employ fewer contract personnel and their activities involve more direct interaction with the public.

Two of the source categories deserve some explanation. The source category designation of "NRC" is used when an NRC staff member suspects a regulatory requirement has been violated deliberately or due to careless disregard, prompting the initiation of an investigation by the NRC Office of Investigations. The source category of "Licensee" is applied in similar circumstances wherein a licensee representative, acting in their official capacity, reports a potential wrongdoing matter to the NRC. An allegation process tracking number is assigned to

---

[4]Few concerns were received from sources representing the 1 percent not depicted in Figure 4. These sources include Federal Agency and State Agency.

such items so that the staff can track the progress of efforts to review the potential wrongdoing issue.

Allegation Trends for Selected Reactor Sites

As noted previously, the trending of allegations received concerning individual reactor sites is one method the NRC staff uses to monitor the safety conscious work environment at reactor sites. Statistics on allegations received concerning all operating reactor sites are provided in a table in Appendix 1. The allegations in the table cover the 5-year period January 2001 through December 2005 and include allegations received from onsite sources only; that is, allegations from current or former licensee employees, current or former contractor employees, or anonymous allegers. For the purpose of this analysis, the NRC assumes anonymous allegations are from onsite personnel.

In determining which reactor sites should receive a more in-depth review, the staff applied the following criteria:

1)   The number of onsite allegations received exceeds 2 times the median value for the reactor industry, but does not exceed three times the median, and there is a 50 percent increase in the number of allegations received over the previous year; or;

2)   The number of onsite allegations received exceeds 3 times the median value.

For CY 2005, the median number of onsite allegations per reactor site was four. The fifteen reactor sites that met one of these criteria are Salem and Hope Creek (23), Browns Ferry Unit 1 (23), Palo Verde Units 1, 2 & 3 (22), Susquehanna Units 1 & 2 (20), St. Lucie Units 1 & 2 (16), Oyster Creek (14), Point Beach Units 1 & 2 (13), Byron Units 1 & 2 (11), Callaway (11), Millstone Units 2 & 3 (10), Sequoyah Units 1 & 2 (10), Seabrook (9), Shearon Harris Units 1 & 2 (9), Dresden Units 2 & 3 (9), and Comanche Peak Units 1 & 2 (9). The first seven sites listed exceeded 3 times the industry median, while the remaining sites exceeded 2 times the median and experienced more than a 50 percent increase in the number of allegations concerning the site. In summary, the trends either do not suggest a weakening safety conscious work environment or the licensee is taking steps to address trends and the NRC is monitoring those activities. A more detailed discussion of each of the sites follows.

Salem and Hope Creek

NRC receipt of allegations concerning Salem and Hope Creek trended upward in 2005 from an already high level in 2004, indicating continuing issues in the SCWE area. While the facilities addressed significant SCWE findings identified in 2003-2004, additional changes at the facilities in 2005 presented new challenges to SCWE improvement, including the licensee's entrance into a Nuclear Operating Services Contract with Exelon in the first quarter, numerous senior management changes on site, and the

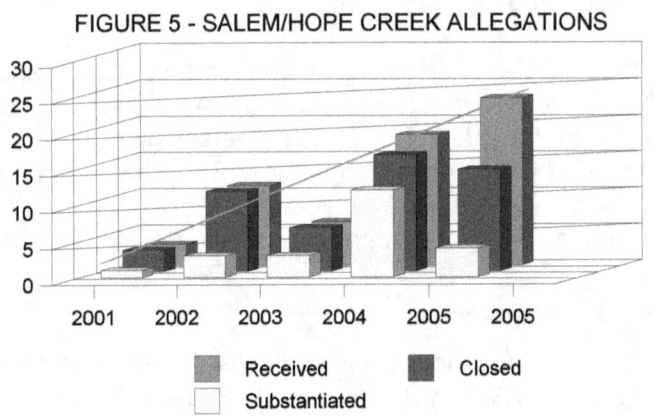

FIGURE 5 - SALEM/HOPE CREEK ALLEGATIONS

implementation of initiatives to address long-standing performance problems. The licensee's inconsistent use of the Executive Review Board process early in 2005, the numerous management changes, and worker uncertainty about the pending merger with Exelon contributed to a range of worker perceptions regarding the advisability of raising issues or challenging decisions.

In the 2005 mid-cycle assessment for Salem and Hope Creek, the staff documented a substantive cross-cutting issue in the SCWE area based on the results of the NRC's ongoing review of the work environment. As a result, Salem and Hope Creek will remain under enhanced NRC oversight per the Reactor Oversight Program Deviation Memorandum dated July 29, 2005, which was renewed to closely monitor the licensee's actions to address issues associated with SCWE. It should be noted that a substantive cross-cutting issue in Problem Identification and Resolution (PI&R) was closed in early 2006 after actions taken by the licensee to improve the resolution of concerns proved effective.

By mid-year, the number of allegations coming to the NRC tapered off and in September 2005, the staff completed a SCWE inspection at the site which concluded that progress has been made in addressing work environment issues. The SCWE inspection team noted some issues that require additional action and focused attention. Specifically, the team identified that, while the licensee had recognized that there was a wide range of perceptions concerning the work environment, they had not taken actions to address and resolve the negative perceptions in the Operations organization in a timely manner. Near-term follow-up actions by the licensee include, plans to implement actions in response to the NRC SCWE inspection report, (IR 05000272/2005013, 05000311/2005013, and 05000354/2005013), conduct a survey of the work environment, perform a self-assessment of SCWE, and provide the results of these efforts to the NRC.

There were five allegations of discrimination at Salem and Hope Creek in 2005. One of these is still under investigation, two were not investigated because the concerned individuals declined to participate in an NRC investigation, and two did not meet the requirements for initiation of an investigation. In order for the NRC to pursue a matter of potential discrimination, pursuant to 10 CFR 50.7, a certain pattern of facts, called a prima-facie showing, must be articulated. Specifically, it must be initially established that an employee has engaged in a protected activity, that an adverse personnel action was taken against the employee, that management knew that the employee had engaged in the protected activity, and that the protected activity was, in part, a reason for the adverse personnel action. In the previous four years (2001 through 2004), nine allegations of discrimination were raised. Two of these were closed because a prima facie showing of potential discrimination was not articulated, and although the remaining seven were investigated, none were substantiated.

In summary, the NRC intends to maintain its enhanced oversight of the SCWE at Salem and Hope Creek until a licensee self-assessment has concluded that substantial, sustainable progress has been made, and the NRC has completed a review, the results of which confirm the licensee's assessment results.

Browns Ferry Unit 1

The number of allegations at Browns Ferry, Unit 1, while high in comparison to the industry median, has remained fairly steady from 2004 to 2005. The number of allegations increased in 2003 coincident with plant construction activities.

Unit 1 of the Browns Ferry site is under construction and has a significant number of contractors on site. The majority of concerns received are consistent with the type of issues expected at a plant under construction, in that they involve the training of individuals performing work or specific maintenance issues. Almost half of the allegations received involved health physics concerns related to one circumstance. The licensee also noted that the issues received internally were consistent with concerns typical of a plant under construction and the increase in health physics issues. In

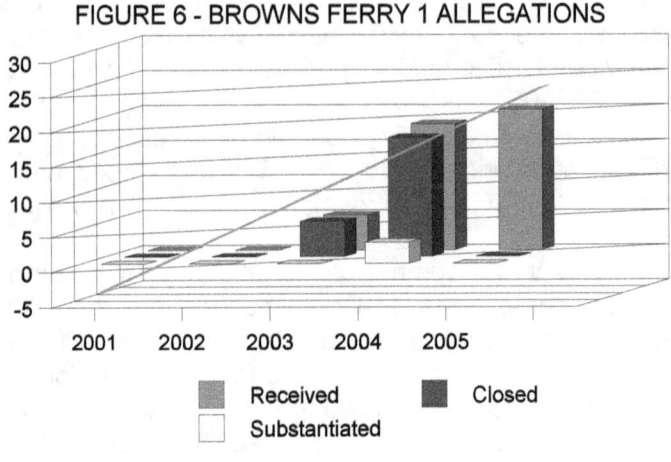

FIGURE 6 - BROWNS FERRY 1 ALLEGATIONS

response to the increase in health physics issues raised internally, the licensee trained its contractor on the as-low-as-is-reasonably-achievable concept in late 2005.

The licensee has taken a number of steps to monitor the SCWE. These included providing SCWE training for contractor personnel, performing assessments of the safety conscious work environment, and implementing program improvements such as assignment of a new Organizational and Cultural Manager to oversee the Employee Concerns Program (ECP). The licensee's Office of the Inspector General completes a SCWE assessment of all of the TVA sites every other year. The assessment in 2004 showed an improvement in the safety conscious work environment with regard to individuals' willingness to raise concerns and their knowledge of the avenues available for raising concerns. However, the assessment indicated that only 73 percent of individuals surveyed at Browns Ferry had confidence that problems on site are resolved. The licensee attributed this less positive result to several issues associated with the corrective action program, including concerns that the threshold for writing corrective action documents was too low, unfamiliarity with the site's new electronic corrective action system, problems with the software upon start up of this new system, perceptions that the root causes of problems were not always addressed, and a perception that corrective action documents are written in a punitive manner, including naming individuals involved in problems identified. In response to this information, the licensee has taken actions to provide information to employees on the type of issue and information that is not appropriate for entry into the corrective action system, address the software issues associated with the electronic corrective action system, and communicate information regarding the purpose and changes to the corrective action system.

In the past three years, there has been an increasing number of allegations of discrimination received. However, the results of investigations performed in response to these issues has not substantiated that discrimination occurred. Of the three discrimination allegations received in 2004, two were withdrawn by the concerned individual and one was investigated, but not substantiated. Of the four received in 2005, two are still ongoing and one was withdrawn by the concerned individual. The licensee noted a slight decrease in the number of discrimination complaints raised internally in 2005.

The nature of allegations received, the lack of a trend in the total number received, along with the volume of concerns being raised internally, do not indicate a weakening SCWE. However, the NRC will continue to monitor the work environment through normal inspection activities, including a review of the actions the licensee takes to improve it, and the general allegation trends at the Browns Ferry Unit 1 site.

Palo Verde Units 1, 2 & 3

The number of allegations from onsite sources concerning the Palo Verde site increased to its highest level in the last five years. An increasing trend in engineering-related concerns was evident in the issues raised. However, the NRC does not believe the increased number of allegations represents a SCWE concern given that several of the issues were very similar in nature and were from a small number of allegers. The licensee's Employee Concerns Program also saw an increase in the number of concerns raised in 2005, although not as significant as the increase in allegations and mostly attributed by the licensee to the unique activities related to steam generator replacements late in the year.

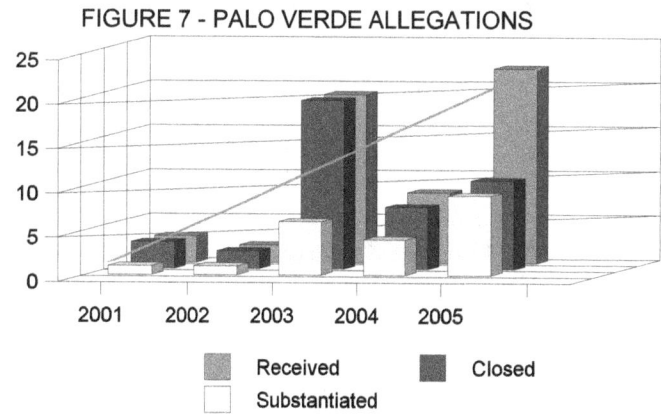

FIGURE 7 - PALO VERDE ALLEGATIONS

The licensee, Arizona Public Service (APS), has taken several actions to monitor and maintain a healthy SCWE at Palo Verde. In the first quarter of 2005, APS commissioned an independent assessment and survey of the safety culture and safety conscious work environment. In August 2005, the NRC met publically with APS to discuss the results of the survey. The results indicate the workforce believed the SCWE was "very good to excellent." A significant percentage of employees indicated they would raise safety concerns to their supervisor or write a condition report and, if unsatisfied with the response, escalate the matter up the chain of command. Additionally, very few indicated they were aware of any negative reactions to employees raising concerns. According to the licensee, leadership training in safety culture and SCWE principles was also recently completed.

There have been no substantiated allegations of discrimination during this review period. Four claims were made in 2005, all of which are still open. Five allegations of discrimination were made between the years 2001 and 2004. All were investigated but the agency did not find sufficient evidence to substantiate the discrimination as alleged.

Although Palo Verde has a high number of allegations, the trends do not suggest a weakening SCWE; neither do the results of the licensee's 2005 independent evaluation of the safety culture and SCWE. The NRC will continue to monitor, through its normal inspection, investigation, and allegation review processes, the SCWE at Palo Verde.

Susquehanna Units 1 & 2

Although NRC receipt of allegations regarding Susquehanna trended downward from 2001 through 2003, the number of allegations increased significantly in 2004 and continued an

upward trend in 2005. While review of individual allegation issues prior to mid-2005 found no particular pattern or trend in the disciplines involved, numerous issues received in the latter half of 2005 highlighted outage maintenance support activities. NRC follow-up efforts with regard to this area are in progress.

In the Fall of 2004, the licensee conducted an independent review of the effectiveness of their ECP. The contractor found that although the program effectively addresses employee concerns, it does not always recognize the potential impact

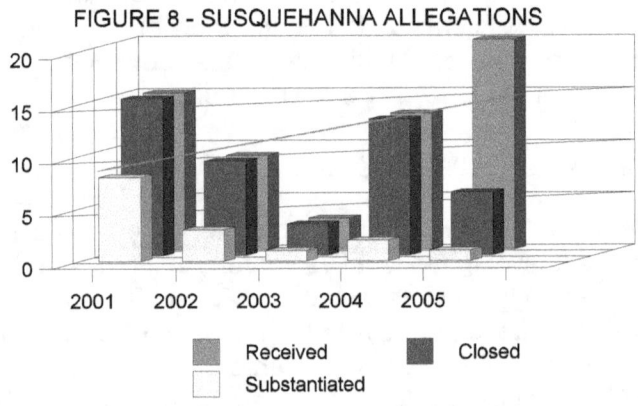

FIGURE 8 - SUSQUEHANNA ALLEGATIONS

management actions may have on the work environment and recommended a number of enhancements. Follow-up actions from that assessment were completed in 2005, including a revision of company policy and communications reinforcing the licensee's commitment to SCWE, presentations to work groups by ECP, improved supervisory training, and expansion of responsibilities for the Employee Concerns Oversight Team. SCWE surveys have been conducted by the licensee at Susquehanna periodically since 1997, and most recently in 2003. The licensee has been addressing issues noted in the maintenance and design engineering areas during the 2003 SCWE survey, and is continuing to address more recent issues in the maintenance area resulting from scheduling and assignment changes. Another SCWE survey will be conducted later in 2006 to assess the effectiveness of actions taken. The licensee also intends to use outside consultants with SCWE expertise to examine the work environment within certain work groups at Susquehanna, including Maintenance.

There were six allegations of discrimination filed in 2005 at Susquehanna. One of these was closed because a prima facie showing of potential discrimination was not articulated, one is currently under investigation, and one is in the Early-ADR process. The three remaining allegations of discrimination were received late in 2005, and were in the early stages of review when this report was written. In the previous four years (2001 through 2004), ten allegations of discrimination were raised. Five of these were closed because a prima facie showing of potential discrimination was not articulated, and although the remaining five were investigated, none were substantiated.

The NRC will continue to monitor with interest the licensee's progress with their indicated initiatives and assessments, in an effort to obtain a clearer picture of work environment issues at Susquehanna. Similarly, the willingness of personnel to raise safety concerns will be probed during interviews conducted as part of the ongoing NRC investigations of discrimination allegations at the site.

St. Lucie Units 1 & 2

Although St. Lucie's allegation trend over the past five years is down, the number of allegations from the site increased in 2005 over the previous year. There were some activities on site during 2005 which likely contributed to the noted increase. For example, the licensee completed two refueling outages, and, during the fall outage, the licensee replaced the reactor vessel head and pressurizer head, which were both significant and unique activities. In addition, a union contract was voted down during 2005. An increase in the number of concerns raised through the ECP and to the NRC coincided with the fall outage.

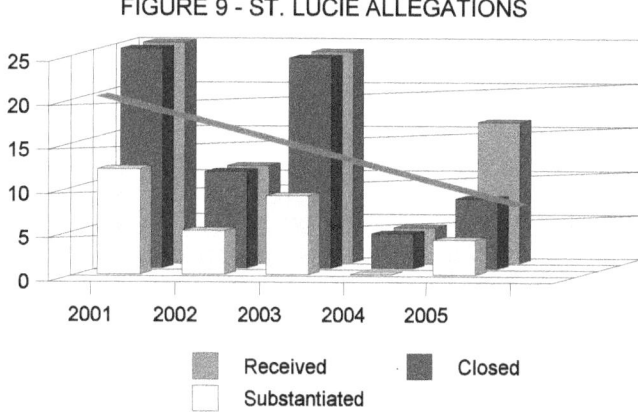

FIGURE 9 - ST. LUCIE ALLEGATIONS

Received   Closed   Substantiated

A review of the allegations received in 2005 indicated that approximately a fifth of the concerns received related to the willingness of employees to raise concerns. However, a review of the actual content of the concerns did not indicate a specific SCWE-related trend that concerns the NRC; that is, since the concerns involved very isolated incidents or narrowly focused issues they did not represent a broader SCWE issue. The NRC also received several allegations regarding security. To ensure that we are not unnecessarily releasing information that would reveal any potential security-related vulnerabilities, the NRC staff is not at liberty to discuss specific information concerning actions taken by the agency or licensee in the security area. The NRC and licensee have taken all necessary actions to address potential security-related concerns that may have been identified during the course of the NRC's review of these allegations. The licensee similarly noted a slight increase in the number of concerns raised internally through the ECP and the Corrective Action Program, and many of these concerns were in the area of security.

In response to an NRC-identified concern with the plant's SCWE in late 2003, the licensee initiated several actions to measure and improve the work environment on site, including restructuring the organization, monitoring the SCWE annually using survey tools, providing SCWE training, enhancing the corrective action program, and initiating a Leadership Development Academy. The licensee indicated that there was evidence of an improving SCWE in 2004. A 2004 PI&R inspection (IR 05000335/2004007 and 05000389/2004007) conducted by the NRC staff similarly did not identify any reluctance by the plant staff to report safety concerns. In 2005, the NRC staff reviewed the effectiveness of the ECP and Corrective Action Program in dealing with SCWE issues (IR 05000335/2005003 and 05000389/2005003). In general, the NRC found that the SCWE at the St. Lucie plant appeared to be healthy and employees felt free to raise issues to their management without fear of retaliation, the licensee's ECP organization was effective in investigating and facilitating the resolution of employee concerns and appropriately addressed individual's concerns, and the licensee was timely in responding to employee concerns with the appropriate prioritization placed on the safety significance of the issue.

The licensee's annual SCWE survey in August 2005 indicated that some individuals may be reluctant to raise concerns through one or more of the methods available and, in particular, the condition reporting system was identified as an area of concern by the workforce. In response, the licensee implemented a new electronic reporting system, established a performance improvement department which monitors the Corrective Action Program's effectiveness, and completed training on the new program. The purpose of the training was to ensure that employees have an understanding of how management prioritizes issues raised based on their safety significance.

The licensee indicated that SCWE issues remain in some organizations on site, and that in many cases these issues resulted from management styles that were not conducive to a healthy SCWE. During 2004 and 2005, senior licensee management emphasized the importance of a healthy SCWE, through supervisory development training and reorganization or removal of supervisors when necessary.

The number of discrimination allegations received over the last five years has remained fairly steady. In 2005, there were four allegations of discrimination filed. One was not substantiated and three were still being investigated at the time this report was written. In 2004, there were three allegations of discrimination raised. Of these three, concerned individuals in two of the cases withdrew their allegations, and one was investigated, but not substantiated. Between 2001 and 2003, there were six discrimination allegations filed; all were investigated, but none were substantiated.

The similarity in the number and nature of concerns raised internally and externally and the timing of the receipt of these concerns with significant and unique onsite activities indicates that the increase noted in 2005 was likely not the result of a decline in the SCWE. However, recognizing that isolated SCWE issues exist in certain organizations on site, the NRC will continue to monitor the work environment at the St. Lucie site to assess the effectiveness of the licensee's recent actions and take further regulatory actions if necessary.

Oyster Creek

Although the volume of allegations concerning the Oyster Creek experienced a 50 percent drop from 2003 to 2004, an increase in 2005 from the prior year was noted. A review of the individual issues received in 2005 found no particular pattern or trend in the disciplines involved.

There were two allegations of discrimination in 2005 concerning activities at Oyster Creek. One is under investigation, and one is in the Early-ADR process. Eight allegations of discrimination were raised at Oyster Creek from 2001 to 2004. Six of the eight were closed because a prima facie showing of potential discrimination was not articulated. The other two discrimination issues were investigated, but not substantiated.

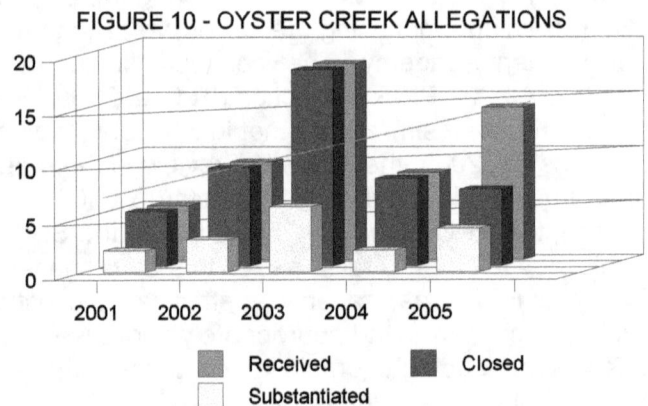

FIGURE 10 - OYSTER CREEK ALLEGATIONS

Received   Closed
Substantiated

The licensee, Exelon, performed a self-assessment of the ECPs across the Exelon Fleet, including Oyster Creek, in 2005. The self-assessment looked at licensee employee and contractor familiarity with ECP, the categorization of concerns received, ECP issue trending and follow-up, and corrective action effectiveness. Results of the self-assessment with regard to Oyster Creek were positive. A SCWE self-assessment is scheduled to be conducted at Oyster Creek in June 2006.

The NRC will continue to monitor the safety conscious work environment through its normal inspection and oversight processes. The NRC will also monitor the actions the licensee takes to improve the work environment as well as the general allegation trend at the Oyster Creek site.

Point Beach Units 1 & 2

The volume of allegations received concerning the Point Beach site reflects a slightly increasing trend over the past five years. Discussions with the licensee identified that, while the number of allegations increased in 2005, concerns raised via the licensee's ECP declined by approximately 40 percent. A review of the issues raised in the 2005 allegations indicates a number of the concerns were related to weaknesses in the SCWE, in that they involved either claims of discrimination, a chilling effect of the environment for raising concerns internally, or concerns about the effectiveness of the Corrective Action Program. The NRC staff identified a substantive cross-cutting issue in the area of PI&R in 2002 and subsequent assessment periods. The licensee's commitments to

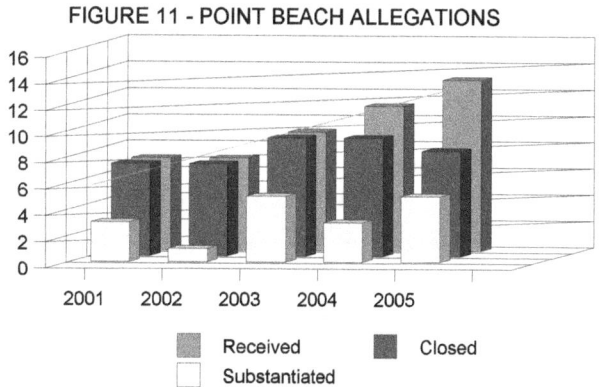

FIGURE 11 - POINT BEACH ALLEGATIONS

make sustained improvements were documented in an NRC Confirmatory Action Letter (CAL) dated April 21, 2004. A review of the licensee's actions recently concluded that the licensee had made progress on most of the CAL commitments and the NRC determined in the most recent annual assessment that the PI&R substantive cross-cutting issue would be closed.

The NRC's evaluation of the SCWE during the 2004 PI&R inspections (IR 05000266/2004008, 05000301/2004008) and 2005 (IR 05000266/2005012, 05000301/2005012), determined that workers at the site felt free to input nuclear safety concerns into the Corrective Action Program. However, the NRC noted that an independent safety culture assessment in mid-2004 and a survey of the workforce commissioned by the licensee in late 2004 identified that some workers did not trust management's ability to appropriately address issues raised. Actions taken in response to the CAL and the mid-year assessment, prior to the results of the survey being known, were designed to improve 1) site leadership behaviors related to safety culture and SCWE, 2) the prioritization of site initiatives, and 3) communication of operational decisions. The licensee expects these actions to also address the declining trust issues identified in the most recent survey. The survey also characterized a number of specific departments on site that warranted near-term management attention due to their significantly lower SCWE ratings and declining trends. The NRC reviewed the actions taken by the licensee during the 2005 PI&R inspection. The inspectors provided the observation that the licensee's actions regarding increased management attention fell short of that called for by the survey's independent assessor.

On March 23, 2006, the staff held a public meeting with the licensee to further discuss actions taken or planned for these specific departments and general work environment. The licensee again described the general actions mentioned above, but provided no information specific to the departments identified with declining SCWE trends during the meeting. The NRC is aware that leadership assessments conducted by the licensee resulted in the coaching or replacing of some supervisors in these departments. Training described by the licensee to improve leadership behaviors related to safety culture and SCWE has not yet been completed. Shortly after the public meeting, the licensee told the NRC it would conduct another survey early in the summer 2006 to assess the effectiveness of their corrective actions. The NRC will review the survey's findings and licensee's actions to address the findings during the normal inspection process.

The NRC also saw an increasing trend with regard to allegations of discrimination. Five discrimination allegations were raised in 2005, two of which were not investigated because a prima-facie showing of potential discrimination was not articulated, and three of which are still open. Of the three allegations of discrimination raised in 2004, two are still open and one was investigated and not substantiated. Between 2001 and 2003, six discrimination claims were made, four of which were investigated but not substantiated and two which did not make a prima-facie showing.

The NRC continues to closely monitor the SCWE at the Point Beach site, including the ongoing investigations of discrimination allegations and the licensee's actions to address the SCWE-related findings identified in the 2004 survey, and will continue to take additional actions if warranted.

Byron Units 1 & 2

Although allegations concerning the Byron site have trended down for several years, in 2005 the trend reversed itself. A review of the individual issues found no pattern or trend in the disciplines involved that would indicate a significant weakness in the SCWE. Similarly, the licensee indicated that the number of concerns going to their ECP increased significantly in 2005. The licensee's Nuclear Safety Review Board questioned the increase and management took actions to improve communications to the workforce concerning events and decisions thought to have contributed to the increased concerns. After an increase particularly in the first two quarters of the year, concerns to the ECP trended down during the remainder of the year. A Fall 2005 licensee initiated self-assessment of the ECP resulted in actions to improve workforce understanding of the licensee's SCWE policy at Byron, and other Exelon sites.

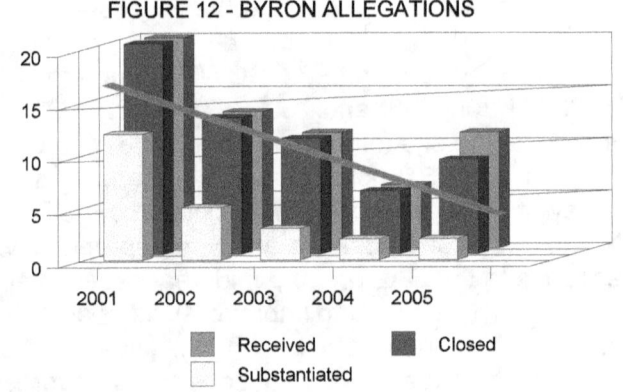

FIGURE 12 - BYRON ALLEGATIONS

The NRC assessed the health of the SCWE during the June 2005 PI&R inspection (IR 05000454/2005008, 05000455/2005008) and found that workers expressed no concerns about identifying issues, and felt comfortable discussing them with supervision without fear of reprisal. The team also observed that all personnel interviewed were aware of the different avenues through which they could express concerns including the Corrective Action Program, informing their supervisor or plant managers, contacting the ECP coordinator, or coming to the NRC;

however, many workers said they preferred reporting issues directly to their immediate supervisor. Workers were generally familiar with the ECP and expressed no concerns with utilizing it.

Three allegations of discrimination were raised in 2005. One was settled between the parties without NRC investigation using the NRC's Early-ADR Program. The other two remain open and under investigation. In 2001, a discrimination allegation was substantiated by the NRC. Corrective actions by the licensee were comprehensive and taken fleet-wide. Regarding the intervening three years, four discrimination allegations were raised. In 2004, the alleger did not articulate a prima-facie case and the concern could not be investigated. The allegation raised in 2003 was investigated but not substantiated. Of the two allegations raised in 2002 neither was investigated; one did not make a prima facie showing and the other was a third-hand complaint of suspected retaliation. The NRC does not pursue third-party complaints due to the lack of specific information about the alleged act and permission from the individual named to release his/her name to the licensee.

The NRC will monitor the open investigations into the claims of discrimination and continue to monitor trends in the allegation data for indications of a weakening safety conscious work environment.

Callaway

The number of concerns received regarding the site increased significantly from 2004 to 2005. The licensee noted a similar increase in the number of concerns raised internally through the ECP. Trending of the allegations received indicated that the majority of the concerns related to security. To ensure that we are not unnecessarily releasing information that would reveal any potential security-related vulnerabilities, the NRC staff is not at liberty to discuss specific information concerning actions taken by the agency or licensee in the security area. The NRC and licensee have taken all necessary actions to address potential security-related concerns that may have been identified during the course of the NRC's review of these allegations. The licensee similarly noted that many of the concerns raised internally related to security. The licensee noted that in 2005, the security force at the site voted in a labor union and that contract negotiations to date have not been successful. These negotiations may have contributed to the increase in allegations noted.

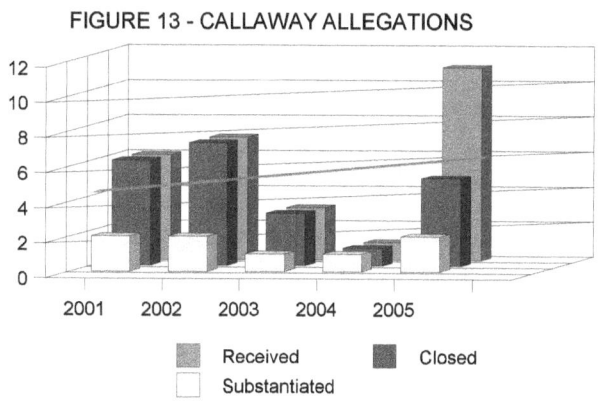

FIGURE 13 - CALLAWAY ALLEGATIONS

In addition to contract negotiations in the security force, the licensee noted that in the fall of 2005, a major outage was conducted during which four steam generators and several low and high pressure turbine rotors were replaced. These major and unique activities likely impacted the number of concerns raised internally. Additionally, in 2005 the Board of Directors tasked the current plant management with improving plant performance. As part of this effort, several senior managers on site were replaced and expectations and accountability of the plant staff have been increased. The change in management, higher expectations regarding the need to identify and resolve safety issues, and some anxiety regarding the changes may have impacted the number of allegations received by the NRC.

The number of discrimination complaints also indicates an increasing trend, with the number increasing from 0 in 2004 to four in 2005. Of the discrimination concerns received in 2005, one was settled through the NRC's Early-ADR pilot process, and three are still being evaluated by the NRC. Between 2001 and 2003, there were three allegations which included a claim of discrimination, one in each of the three years. None of these allegations were substantiated.

The licensee indicated that in the last few years, significant emphasis has been placed on improving the visibility of the ECP and establishing a SCWE. For example, since 2003, the licensee has developed a website for the ECP, incorporated SCWE concepts and expectations into supervisory skills training, and provided briefings regarding the SCWE for contractors working on site. The most recent PI&R inspection conducted by the NRC staff in May 2004 indicated that most individuals were aware of the changes to the program (IR 05000483/2004006). The licensee attributes a noted increase in the number of concerns raised internally both through the ECP and in condition reporting, to these efforts. The licensee also noted a decreasing trend in the number of corrective action documents filed anonymously, which indicates that individuals feel free to document issues without fear of retaliation.

During the NRC's PI&R inspection, the NRC staff concluded that a SCWE exists at the site. However, some negative comments regarding confidence in the Corrective Action Program were made during interviews. The NRC did determine in 2004 that a cross-cutting issue in the area of PI&R existed. However, since that time, the NRC has determined that the licensee has taken sufficient actions to address the issues related to PI&R, such as revising the methodology for conducting root causes and the threshold for initiating problem reports. As a result, the cross-cutting issue was closed. A recent assessment conducted by the NRC (IR 05000483/2006002) concluded that further improvements in the area of corrective actions were needed, but that the licensee had made significant improvements.

The licensee had a site survey conducted by an independent contractor in May 2005. The results of the survey demonstrated that workforce perceptions of the SCWE and ECP had improved significantly. The employee concerns staff provided recommendations to address specific issues in some departments following the survey. The licensee attributes the improvement to changes in site senior management and efforts to address equipment reliability and human performance issues. The new management team continues to emphasize accountability and increased standards, and the licensee has noted some concerns internally related to this increased accountability.

The similarity in the type and number of concerns raised internally and externally, the site activities which likely contributed to the noted increase in the number of allegations received by the NRC, and improvements noted in the SCWE as a result of the recent independent survey results indicate that the increase in allegations noted does not represent a decline in the site's safety conscious work environment. However, the NRC staff will continue to monitor allegation trends, efforts taken by the licensee to improve the SCWE, and results of the site's SCWE assessments for insights into the work environment at Callaway.

Millstone Units 2 & 3

There was a significant increase in allegations regarding Millstone in 2005, primarily in the security area. To ensure that the NRC is not unnecessarily releasing information that would reveal any potential security related vulnerabilities, the NRC staff is not at liberty to discuss specific information concerning actions taken by the agency or licensee in the security area. The NRC and licensee have taken all necessary actions to address potential security-related concerns that have been identified during the course of the NRC's review of these allegations. The licensee has acknowledged the increasing level of concern from onsite sources in the security area.

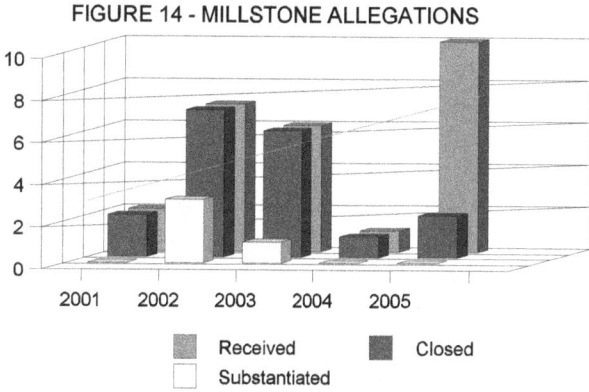

FIGURE 14 - MILLSTONE ALLEGATIONS

Received   Closed
Substantiated

There were six allegations of discrimination in 2005 concerning activities at Millstone. All six are still under investigation, and several are interrelated. The state of Connecticut (Attorney General and Department of Public Utility Control) has shown an interest in some of the discrimination cases and is conducting its own investigation of at least one alleged discrimination case. Four allegations of discrimination were raised at Millstone from 2001 - 2004 (three in 2002 and one in 2004). Of the three discrimination allegations raised in 2002, one was investigated and not substantiated, and the others were not investigated because a prima facie assertion of discrimination was not articulated. The alleger in 2004 was also determined not to have articulated a prima facie assertion of discrimination.

An analysis of the trends in allegations does not suggest a SCWE problem at Millstone. The licensee continues to monitor their work environment using survey tools. A facility-wide culture survey was conducted in late 2004 and identified no areas of concern. Another culture survey is planned for late 2006. The staff will continue to monitor the general trend of allegations, particularly in the security area. The staff will also continue to monitor trends in the licensee's internal reporting programs through normal inspection and oversight processes, as well as the open discrimination case files.

Sequoyah Units 1 & 2

The number of allegations at Sequoyah has been relatively steady over the review period and has remained near the median number for operating power reactors. However, from 2004 to 2005 there was a notable increase in the number received. No trend was noted in the 2005 allegation data. The licensee also noted an increase in the number of concerns raised through the site's employee concerns program. Most of the issues received internally were reported during the site's spring outage; the number of concerns received by the NRC similarly increased

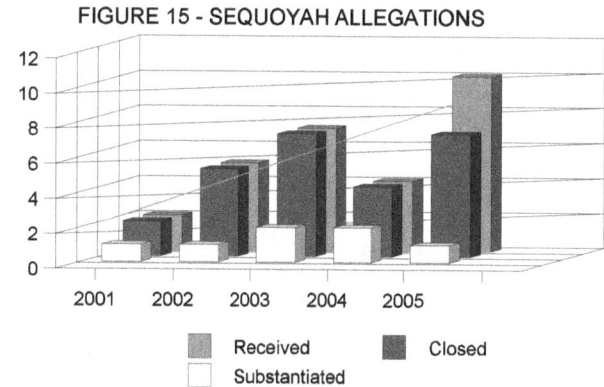

FIGURE 15 - SEQUOYAH ALLEGATIONS

Received   Closed
Substantiated

coincident with the spring outage. The number of condition reports generated by site employees has remained relatively constant.

Contacts with NRC regional staff and the site indicate that no unusual activities occurred on site which may have contributed to the increase in allegations in 2005. None of the performance deficiencies identified during the NRC's baseline inspection program had cross-cutting aspects in the areas of SCWE or PI&R as it relates to willingness to raise concerns.

As discussed under Browns Ferry Unit 1 above, the licensee's Office of the Inspector General completes a SCWE assessment of all of its sites every other year. The last assessment, conducted in 2004, did not identify significant problems. The survey indicated that employees at Sequoyah would raise safety concerns and that they knew what venues were available to them for raising concerns. Slightly fewer employees, however, believed that the licensee was resolving safety issues that were raised. The corrective actions described for Browns Ferry Unit 1 were also taken at the Sequoyah plant in response to these findings. The licensee has also created a position for organizational cultural initiatives that reports to the company Chief Nuclear Officer and oversees the licensee's efforts with regard to the ECP. The licensee is planning to conduct a safety culture assessment in May 2006 to assess the effectiveness of actions taken improve the SCWE.

The lack of a trend in the types of allegations received and the timing of the issues received indicates that there is not a concern with a weakening SCWE. The NRC will continue to monitor the number and nature of allegations received as well as the results of the upcoming SCWE assessments during normal inspection activities to further evaluate the safety conscious work environment.

Seabrook

There was a noted increase in allegations regarding Seabrook in 2005, primarily in the security area. The licensee also had some similar concerns raised internally. To ensure that the NRC is not unnecessarily releasing information that would reveal any potential security-related vulnerabilities, the NRC staff is not at liberty to discuss specific information concerning actions taken by the agency or the licensee in the security area. The NRC and licensee have taken all necessary actions to address potential security-related concerns that have been identified during the course of the NRC's review of these allegations. The licensee has acknowledged and is addressing the increasing level of concern from onsite sources in the security area.

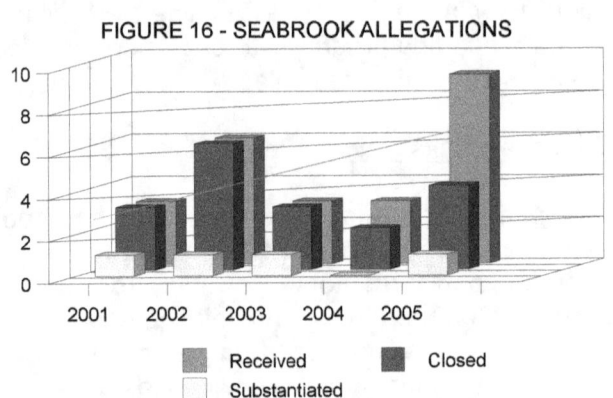

FIGURE 16 - SEABROOK ALLEGATIONS

There were three allegations of discrimination in 2005 concerning activities at Seabrook. All are still under investigation. Two allegations of discrimination were raised at Seabrook from 2001 to 2004. A 2002 discrimination concern was investigated and was not substantiated. In 2004, after review of a Department of Labor Administrative Law Judge finding of discrimination, the NRC sent "chilling effect letters" to Florida Power and Light (FPL, the licensee for Seabrook) as well as to another affected utility and a contractor, requesting information on any actions planned or taken to mitigate potential impacts of this finding on their respective SCWEs. FPL's November 2004 response to the chilling effect letter emphasized the company's commitment to maintaining a SCWE, and discussed recent initiatives that included training and assessment with regard to SCWE, such as a Leadership Forum/Supervisory Development Academy initiated in 2004, safety culture training provided to FPL Nuclear Division managers in 2003 on lessons learned from the Davis-Besse incident, development of company policy documentation regarding SCWE in December 2004, and conduct of an annual SCWE survey at each FPL plant in October 2005. While the results of the SCWE survey are being independently evaluated, the licensee has taken some actions to gather supporting information from the workforce through focus groups to help structure any actions needed to respond to the findings.

Based on a review of the Office of Investigation's report and DOL documentation related to the 2004 matter, the NRC concluded that the concerned individual voluntarily left a position at the other facility and was not discriminated against in that instance. However, an apparent violation was identified at Seabrook and was considered for escalated enforcement in accordance with the NRC Enforcement Policy. The apparent violation of 10 CFR 50.7, "Employee Protection," involved the individual's de-selection for employment by a contractor at Seabrook, for engaging in a protected activity (for expressing a safety concern at another facility). After taking into consideration that FPL had no knowledge of the decision by the concerned individual's contract employer not to hire him/her, and the actions taken by FPL in response to the chilling effect letter of October 20, 2004, the NRC decided not to pursue enforcement action against the licensee.

An analysis of the trends in allegations does not suggest a SCWE problem at Seabrook. The licensee continues to monitor its work environment through annual SCWE surveys along with SCWE training and guidance provided by other established processes. The NRC will continue to monitor the general trend of allegations through normal inspection and oversight processes, particularly in the security area. The NRC will also monitor trends in the licensee's internal reporting programs, as well as the open discrimination case files at Seabrook.

Shearon Harris Units 1 & 2

The number of allegations at Shearon Harris increased significantly from zero in 2004 to nine in 2005. The number received in 2005 was a significant difference from the number received in any of the last 5 years. The majority of the concerns received were in the area of security. To ensure that we are not unnecessarily releasing information that would reveal any potential security-related vulnerabilities, the NRC staff is not at liberty to discuss specific information concerning actions taken by the agency or the licensee in the security area. The NRC and licensee have taken all necessary actions to address potential security-related concerns that may have been identified during the course of the NRC's review of these allegations.

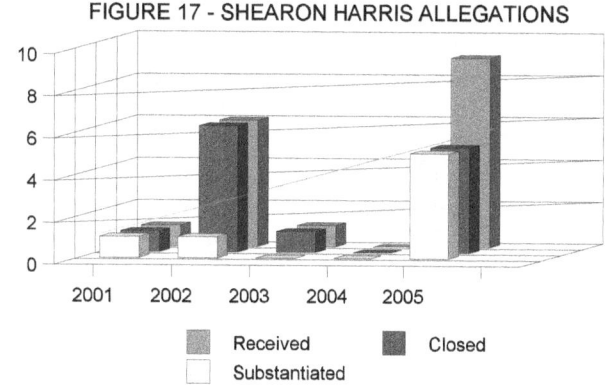

FIGURE 17 - SHEARON HARRIS ALLEGATIONS

The licensee confirmed that they too had seen a notable increase in the volume of concerns raised internally by their employees specifically in the area of security. The similarity of the information indicates that licensee employees were willing to raise issues internally as well as to the NRC. There are a number of factors which may have impacted the increase in the number of allegations at the site. For example, there is an ongoing effort to unionize many positions on site and there was a voluntary reduction in force in 2005. There has also been frequent turnover in security management.

The licensee identified that there was an increase in the number of concerns received internally and externally in the area of security by mid-2005 and, as a result, conducted an assessment of the safety conscious work environment in that department. The licensee assessment indicated actions to improve the SCWE were warranted and the licensee has instituted a plan to address such issues. Discussions with the site indicated that some improvements in the work environment in the security department have been noted, such as a willingness of the security force to interact directly with a newly appointed Project Manager. The NRC recently conducted an inspection of security concerns at Shearon Harris, including issues that involved SCWE. The NRC did not identify widespread reluctance among workers at the plant to raise safety concerns; rather, the issues in the security department related to one type of issue. The licensee took appropriate steps to address this concern.

The number of discrimination concerns has not increased in the last five years. Only one allegation of discrimination has been received in the last five years. That allegation was received in 2002, but later withdrawn at the request of the individual.

The data supports that issues impacting the SCWE in the security department are limited to that department and the NRC found that the issues in the department are related to one type of issue. The licensee is addressing the issues in a proactive manner. The NRC will continue under the normal inspection and oversight processes to monitor allegation trends and the work environment.

Dresden Units 2 & 3

Similar to the trends at Byron, another Exelon site, the allegations concerning the Dresden site have trended down for several years, but in 2005 the trend reversed itself. A review of the issues, however, found no pattern or trend indicating a weakening SCWE site-wide or in any one particular area. Based on discussions with the licensee, the number of concerns raised internally to the licensee's ECP remained steady over the last two calendar years. A Fall 2005 licensee initiated self-assessment of the ECP resulted in actions to improve the visibility of ECP personnel at Dresden, and other Exelon sites.

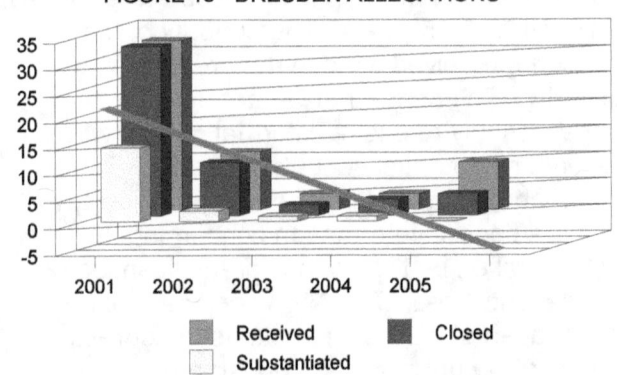

FIGURE 18 - DRESDEN ALLEGATIONS

With regard to allegations of discrimination there was a slight increase in 2005. Three allegations of discrimination were made to the NRC in 2005. Two of the allegations were not investigated because a prima facie showing of discrimination was not articulated. The remaining 2005 discrimination allegation is still open and under investigation. Two allegations of discrimination, one in each year, were raised in 2002 and 2003 and investigated, but the agency did not find sufficient evidence to substantiate the allegation. Nonetheless, the allegations remain open pending conclusion of Department of Labor proceedings on the same cases. There were 10 allegations of discrimination raised at Dresden in 2001; seven of the 10 were investigated by the agency but not substantiated, one did not make a prima facie showing, and two were withdrawn by the concerned individuals. Corrective actions, including conducting SCWE training for supervisory personnel, were taken by the licensee at all its sites, including Dresden, after a finding of discrimination at Byron in 2001.

The NRC will continue to monitor the SCWE at the Dresden site through normal processes, including the ongoing investigations of discrimination allegations, inspections, and allegation program data reviews.

Comanche Peak Units 1 & 2

The number of allegations at the site increased sharply from two to nine from 2004 to 2005. A review of the allegations received indicates that many of the concerns related to technical issues in the Quality Assurance organization and chilling effect allegations in both the Quality Assurance and Operations organizations. The number of discrimination complaints has also risen from zero in the last four years, to three in 2005.

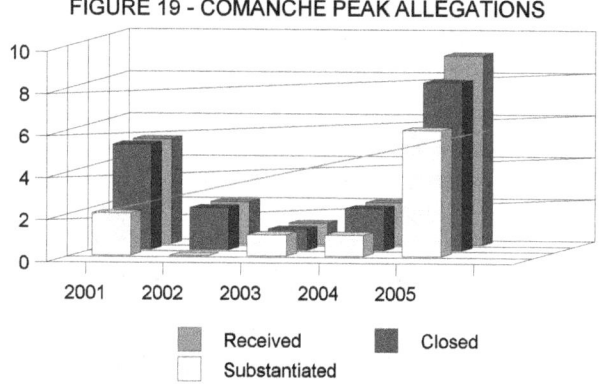

FIGURE 19 - COMANCHE PEAK ALLEGATIONS

The licensee similarly noted an increase in the number of quality assurance issues raised internally. The licensee attributes the issues raised mostly to an audit conducted by the quality assurance group of the procurement quality assurance group within the same organization which created some animosity among the groups. The licensee had recognized the potential impact of this animosity on the SCWE and had completed a cultural survey of the organization in 2005. The survey identified that there were issues of trust and resentment among the staff in the Quality Assurance organization. The licensee continues to take actions to address the work environment in the organization through implementation of a communication plan, completing personality analysis of the individuals in the organization to glean insights about the manner in which those in the organization could work to improve the environment, and emphasizing behavioral expectations.

The licensee had also identified the work environment issues in the Operations department and attributed the issues to a rapid turnover in Operations management over the last few years. The new management has emphasized the importance of using human performance tools and has held individuals accountable for the use of such tools; these changing expectations may have caused some tension among the workforce that was reflected in concerns raised to the NRC. In 2003, the licensee performed a SCWE survey of shift personnel and found a significant percentage of shift operations personnel felt intimidated or discouraged from raising safety issues. A follow-up survey in 2004 indicated marked safety culture and organizational improvements, mostly in the area of management styles, that were more conducive to encouraging raising concerns. However, approximately 30 percent of licensed reactor operators continued to express that they felt intimidated or discouraged from raising safety concerns.

The PI&R inspection conducted by the NRC staff in July 2005 concluded that the licensee had established a SCWE at Comanche Peak (IR 05000455/2005009 and 05000446/2005009). The team determined that employees and contractors felt free to enter issues into the Corrective Action Program and raise safety concerns to their supervision, to the ECP, and to the NRC. All plant personnel interviewed by the team, stated that potential safety issues were addressed by the licensee. However, the licensee had identified long-term organizational effectiveness issues within the Operations department, which continued to challenge the SCWE for shift operations personnel. The team concluded that licensee's past actions to improve the Operations department organizational effectiveness had not been fully effective.

A survey completed by an independent contractor in the fall of 2005 indicated improvements in the overall SCWE at the site and the site was categorized as being in the top quartile of the commercial nuclear power sites in the contractor's database for almost all key cultural metrics. However, the results of the survey reiterate that some SCWE issues exist within the Quality Assurance and Operations organizations. The survey also identified an additional area of focus in the warehouse department, which is responsible for procurement activities. The licensee plans to solicit input from employees in these areas regarding the reasons for their negative responses such that action plans can be developed to address the causes of the work environment issues in these departments.

There is similarity in the areas identified by the NRC staff and the licensee as having challenges to the safety conscious work environment. Actions are continuing to be taken by the licensee to address these issues. The NRC staff will continue to monitor the licensee's actions to improve the safety conscious work environment in areas identified as warranting increased attention.

Allegation Trends for Selected Materials Licensees

Recently the NRC began posting certain fuel cycle facilities' allegation statistics on its website (see Appendix 1). Similar information has been available for reactors for a number of years. But because of the small number of allegations received concerning other smaller materials licensees and because of the potential for a licensee or contractor to identify an alleger, tables of statistics on allegations concerning materials licensees other than fuel cycle facilities have not been provided publically or included in this report. None of the material licensees, fuel cycle facilities or otherwise, received a sufficient number of allegations to discern a trend or pattern, or provide insights into the safety conscious work environment, therefore, more in-depth reviews of specific materials licensees were not performed.

Allegation Trends for Selected Vendors

Because none of the vendors received a sufficient number of allegations to discern a trend or pattern, or provide insights into the work environment, more in-depth reviews of specific vendors were not performed. Statistics by contractor or vendor are not given in this report or otherwise provided publically because publishing the number of allegations received has the potential of identifying an alleger.

CONCLUSIONS

From calendar year 2001 through 2005 the number of allegations received by the NRC has remained steady with incremental annual increases in the reactor area from 2003 to 2005. From a regional perspective, there has been an increase in the number of concerns received for operating power reactors over the last five years in all regions except for Region III. In contrast, the number of materials issues has declined over the five-year period in every region.

The analyses of allegations has provided insights into the SCWE at several facilities. The staff has taken action to engage licensees concerning their work environment where warranted and will continue to monitor these sites with interest. Training to be conducted in 2006 associated with the agency's safety culture initiative will include additional guidance for the NRC inspection staff in this area.

Based on information available to date on the agency's Early-ADR process the staff has concluded that the assumed benefits, including decreased costs and the impact on the SCWE, warrant its continued use in the Allegation Program.

Finally, based on concerns that changes to the process by which the NRC handles security-related allegations have the potential to impact the public's willingness to raise such concerns to the NRC, the staff is working with NSIR to improve guidance concerning the level of detail which can appropriately be provided to allegers.

RECOMMENDATIONS

The Agency Allegations Advisor has no recommendations for program changes at this time.

APPENDIX 1

ALLEGATIONS STATISTICS
OPERATING REACTORS AND FUEL FACILITIES

OPERATING REACTOR ALLEGATIONS RECEIVED FROM ONSITE SOURCES

Site	2001	2002	2003	2004	2005
SALEM/HOPE CREEK	3	11	6	18	23
PALO VERDE 1, 2, & 3	3	2	19	8	22
SUSQUEHANNA 1 & 2	15	9	3	13	20
ST LUCIE 1 & 2	25	11	24	4	16
OYSTER CREEK	5	9	18	8	14
POINT BEACH 1 & 2	7	7	9	11	13
BYRON 1 & 2	20	13	11	6	11
CALLAWAY	6	7	3	1	11
TURKEY POINT 3 & 4	11	2	3	9	10
MILLSTONE 2 & 3	2	7	6	1	10
SAN ONOFRE 2 & 3	7	11	11	13	10
SEQUOYAH 1 & 2	2	5	7	4	10
PILGRIM	3	2	5	14	9
SEABROOK	3	6	3	3	9
INDIAN POINT 2 & 3	17	29	20	19	9
HARRIS 1 & 2	1	6	1		9
DRESDEN 2 & 3	32	11	3	3	9
DAVIS-BESSE	2	27	17	12	9
COMANCHE PEAK 1 & 2	5	2	1	2	9
LIMERICK 1 & 2	2	7	4	4	8
BEAVER VALLEY 1 & 2	7	1	1	9	7
COOK 1 & 2	12	14	9	12	7
GRAND GULF	5	6		6	7
COLUMBIA PLANT	13	5	4	6	7
PEACH BOTTOM 2 & 3	2	1	2	1	5
PRAIRIE ISLAND 1 & 2		5	2	4	5
BROWNS FERRY 2 & 3	2	2		6	5
VOGTLE 1 & 2	1	3	1	1	5
SOUTH TEXAS 1 & 2	4	6	2	6	4
FARLEY 1 & 2	3	1	3	1	4
THREE MILE ISLAND	5	5	1	6	4
ARKANSAS 1 & 2	2	3	4	6	4
NINE MILE POINT 1 & 2	4	5	2	4	4
PALISADES	4	9	7	10	4
BRAIDWOOD 1 & 2	5	5	1	3	4
PERRY	7	5	5	12	4
FITZPATRICK	1	1	7		3
WOLF CREEK	4	1			3
KEWAUNEE	4	3	4	3	3
HATCH 1 & 2	2	3	2	1	3
BRUNSWICK 1 & 2	1	1	3	2	3

Site	2001	2002	2003	2004	2005
OCONEE 1, 2, & 3	5	1	3	11	3
WATTS BAR	4	8	2	4	2
CRYSTAL RIVER	2	2	3	4	2
DIABLO CANYON 1 & 2	6	3	2	2	2
WATERFORD	2	7		1	2
MCGUIRE 1 & 2			2	2	2
QUAD CITIES 1 & 2	1	3	1	1	2
FORT CALHOUN	2	2	3	2	2
RIVER BEND	1	1	4	3	2
GINNA		1	2		2
SURRY 1 & 2	2	4	2	1	2
NORTH ANNA 1 & 2	1	10	1	4	2
MONTICELLO			1		2
FERMI	3	4	2	2	2
LASALLE 1 & 2	2	1	2		2
CLINTON	1	3	2	4	1
ROBINSON	1				1
CALVERT CLIFFS 1 & 2	2	3	4	5	1
DUANE ARNOLD	3	2	2	8	1
COOPER	8	6	8	10	1
VERMONT YANKEE		4		3	1
SUMMER	3	2	4	3	
CATAWBA 1 & 2	7		2	2	

FUEL CYCLE FACILITY ALLEGATIONS RECEIVED FROM ONSITE SOURCES

Site	2001	2002	2003	2004	2005
Framatone-Lynchburg				1	
Framatone-Richland	1		1	1	
Global Nuclear Fuel				1	2
Honeywell		3		2	7
Paducah	32	15	22	10	7
Portsmouth	9	6	2	7	2
Westinghouse				1	8